An End to Off-Again On-Again Diet Merry-Go-Rounds!

HERE IS A NEW, SCIENTIFICALLY TESTED *PERMANENT* METHOD TO TAKE WEIGHT OFF—AND KEEP IT OFF—FOREVER.

With the aid of superbly practical advice, easy-to-follow self-help exercises, psychological "tricks" that really work, inspiring sample menus, and above all a wonderfully effective 7 day self-study program, this book offers THE FIRST HONEST ASSURANCE OF SUCCESS IN *GETTING* SLIM AND *KEEPING* SLIM YOUR WHOLE HAPPY, HEALTHY LIFE LONG!

" 'HOW TO BE A WINNER AT THE WEIGHT LOSS GAME' *IS* A WINNER. IT'S THE BEST AID TO WILLPOWER SINCE COTTAGE CHEESE."

—Peter Passell
author of *The Best*

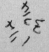

HOW TO BE A WINNER AT THE WEIGHT LOSS GAME

The Behavior Modification Way to Lose Weight and Keep It Off Forever

Walter H. Fanburg, M.D.
Bernard M. Snyder, M.D.

BALLANTINE BOOKS • NEW YORK

Library of Congress Catalog Card Number: 74-29352

ISBN 0-345-24920-8-150

This edition published by arrangement with
Simon & Schuster, New York.

Manufactured in the United States of America

First Ballantine Books Edition: April, 1976

ACKNOWLEDGMENTS

We are indebted to the many people—researchers and those seeking help for overweight who have contributed to the fund of knowledge that has served as a foundation for the development of this book.

Jeanne M. Reid, Research Dietician for the National Institutes of Arthritis, Metabolism, and Digestive Diseases, National Institute of Health, reviewed the nutrition sections of this book; we are most appreciative for her suggestions.

We would like to give special thanks to Patricia Orange for her patience, and superb work on the many changes in the manuscript.

We also give particular thanks to Phyllis Grann, our editor, for her enthusiastic encouragement and expert advice.

TO

EILEEN, DEBBIE, AND JULIE
—WHF

ELAINE, DEBBIE, JONATHAN, AND AARON
—BMS

CONTENTS

PART II
HOW TO CHANGE YOUR EATING BEHAVIOR
AND BE ON YOUR WAY TO PERMANENT
WEIGHT LOSS

PART III
PRACTICING YOUR NEW EATING BEHAVIOR CAN BE FUN AND REWARDING

We advise you to consult your physician before you participate in this or any other weight loss program.

INTRODUCTION

If you haven't been able to lose weight or maintain weight loss, this book is for you. Other approaches have promised you permanent success through various fad diets (some dangerous to your health), pills, gimmicks, etc., but they have all ultimately failed because they overlooked the major problem—your overweight style of eating.

No fad diet and no diet pill can alter your overweight eating habits, because *only you* can change this faulty style. You *can* do it, once you really look at and identify the behavior patterns that make up the way you eat. You have learned patterns of behavior that cause you to overeat. For example, you eat not only when you are hungry, but when you are anxious, angry, or depressed.

Do the following scenes have a familiar ring? You had a fight with your husband—he storms out of the house. Angry and resentful, you rush to the refrigerator and begin gorging yourself. Or you are watching TV. Deeply engrossed in your favorite program, you automatically nibble away at a box of cookies or bag of potato chips without really being aware that you are eating.

To successfully lose weight, you must change your eating behavior, and this book helps you do just that. Our technique puts the emphasis where it belongs: on training you to develop new, healthier eating habits.

In learning a sport like tennis, you must concentrate your efforts on developing a sound stroke. To accomplish this, you identify the components of your present stroke (style) that are faulty, and then substitute new patterns of movement for them. If you practice these new movements, in time you acquire a new, more effective stroke. Practicing a new behavior makes it automatic (it becomes a habit). Just as this process can lead to a winning game of tennis, so too it can lead to successful and permanent weight loss.

Applying this principle to weight loss, you can see how foolish previous advice to "stick to your diet!" has been. It's like telling you to be a better tennis player without showing you how to hit the ball properly. To lose weight and successfully maintain the loss, you must first observe your own troublesome eating behavior. Next you must identify and eliminate those factors that contribute to it. Finally, you must learn and practice new and constructive eating patterns that will bring about the desired weight loss. Through practice, habits are formed which will automatically lead to the desired weight loss and maintenance.

If you follow our simple, step-by-step approach, successful and permanent weight loss can easily be within your reach.

PART I

Look at Your Current
Eating Behavior

Your First Step
to Successful
and
Permanent
Weight Loss

1.

How to Observe Your Eating Behavior

You have your own individual eating style that contributes to your being overweight. In order to become permanently successful at weight loss, you must discover which behavioral patterns in this style are the ones that are troublesome and need to be changed.

To begin, look at your eating style from the following aspects:

1. **What food was taken?**
2. **How much food was eaten?**
3. **How fast was it eaten?**
4. **Where was it eaten?**
5. **What circumstances existed during eating?** (For example, What were your feelings? What else was occurring? Who was present?)

After studying your eating habits, you will become aware of the problem areas. Our book will then show you exactly what to do about them.

You may think that you already know a great deal about your eating behavior, but experience has shown that it is not enough to mentally review the answers to the above questions. You must keep an accurate written record. For example, your record might read as follows: "9:15 AM—argument with boss. I was hurt and furious and gorged myself with candy from the vending machine in the office."

You learn from this kind of observation that eating may occur when you become hurt or angry. Then you will be able to work on other ways to deal with these feelings. For instance, rather than reaching for food, you could reach for the telephone and express your feelings to an understanding friend.

Now you are ready to work on your Eating Behavior Charts, which are found on pages 22–35. Keep them accurately as you eat for the next seven days. Familiarize yourself with the headings across the top of your Eating Behavior Charts:

1. "Eating times"—record the time you *began* eating (1a) and the time you finished (1b).
2. "What was consumed"—record the kind of food eaten (peas, chicken, etc.).
3. "How much?" To help you with weight and volume measures, buy yourself a small food scale. Counting calories can be helpful, but it is important to place the emphasis on your eating behavior.

4. "Place"—this refers to where you eat (dining room, den, bedroom, restaurant, office, coffee shop).
5. "What other activities were occurring?" Were you watching TV, reading a newspaper, or shopping?
6. "Feelings?"—this refers to your emotional state immediately before and during eating. (These might include feelings of anxiety, sadness, happiness, loneliness, or frustration.)
7. "Who was around?" Were you eating alone or with other persons?

TASK NO. 1

Complete the charts on pages 22–35.

Do this in meticulous detail. You are to record every item of food you eat, hour by hour at any time of the day or night.

Make no attempt to alter your present eating behavior.

EATING BEHAVIOR CHART

DAY 1

1 Eating times: Begin Ended a b	2 What was consumed?	3 How much?	4 Place?

5 What other activities were occurring?	6 Feelings?	7 Who was around?	Optional: Caloric value of food consumed?*

Total daily calories consumed _____

* Use any suitable calorie counter.

EATING BEHAVIOR CHART

DAY 2

1 Eating times: Begin Ended a b	2 What was consumed?	3 How much?	4 Place?

5 What other activities were occurring?	6 Feelings?	7 Who was around?	Optional: Caloric value of food consumed?*

Total daily calories consumed _____

* Use any suitable calorie counter.

EATING BEHAVIOR CHART

DAY 3

1 Eating times: Begin Ended a b	2 What was consumed?	3 How much?	4 Place?

5 What other activities were occurring?	6 Feelings?	7 Who was around?	Optional: Caloric value of food consumed?*

Total daily calories consumed _____

* Use any suitable calorie counter.

EATING BEHAVIOR CHART

DAY 4

1 Eating times: Begin Ended a b	2 What was consumed?	3 How much?	4 Place?

5 What other activities were occurring?	6 Feelings?	7 Who was around?	Optional: Caloric value of food consumed?*

Total daily calories consumed _____

* Use any suitable calorie counter.

EATING BEHAVIOR CHART

DAY 5

1 Eating times: Begin Ended a b	2 What was consumed?	3 How much?	4 Place?

5 What other activities were occurring?	6 Feelings?	7 Who was around?	Optional: Caloric value of food consumed?*

Total daily calories consumed _____

* Use any suitable calorie counter.

EATING BEHAVIOR CHART

DAY 6

1 Eating times: Begin Ended a b	2 What was consumed?	3 How much?	4 Place?

5 What other activities were occurring?	6 Feelings?	7 Who was around?	Optional: Caloric value of food consumed?*

Total daily calories consumed _____

* Use any suitable calorie counter.

EATING BEHAVIOR CHART

DAY 7

1 Eating times: Begin a Ended b	2 What was consumed?	3 How much?	4 Place?

5 What other activities were occurring?	6 Feelings?	7 Who was around?	Optional: Caloric value of food consumed?*

Total daily calories consumed _____

* Use any suitable calorie counter.

2.

Evaluating Your
Eating Behavior

Now that you have completed the seven daily eating behavior charts you are ready to study them in detail.

---

1. Are You Eating Too Fast?

Look at column 1 of your Eating Behavior Charts. Record the number of minutes it took to consume the food in the spaces below.

	Breakfast	Lunch	Dinner	Snacks
Day 1				
Day 2				
Day 3				
Day 4				
Day 5				
Day 6				
Day 7				
TOTALS				

Divide by 7

At the bottom of each column, total the time for your main meals and divide by 7, giving the average time spent for breakfast, lunch, and dinner. In addition, add up the number of minutes for all snacks and then divide by the number of snack periods to arrive at your average snack time per day.

TASK NO. 2

Draw in the number of minutes on the clock faces for the average amount of time engaged in eating:

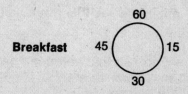

37

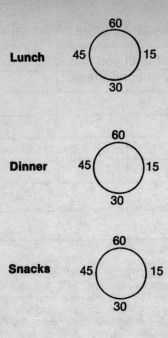

Lunch

60
45 15
30

Dinner

60
45 15
30

Snacks

60
45 15
30

Answer the following questions about how fast you consume food:

1. Do you eat your meals in less than 20 to 30 minutes?

2. Do you put more food in your mouth before swallowing?

3. Do you eat so fast that you don't give yourself time to taste or appreciate your food?

4. Do you frequently finish before others?

5. Do you eat until you feel full and then later feel physically uncomfortable?

If the answer to any of the above questions is yes, you have a problem—*you eat too fast!*

TASK NO. 3

Check the answer to the questions

	Yes	**No**
1.	_____	_____
2.	_____	_____
3.	_____	_____
4.	_____	_____
5.	_____	_____

2. Are You Satisfying Your Nutritional Needs?

The following foods provide you with sufficient protein, carbohydrates, fats, vitamins, and minerals for a healthy, well-balanced diet:

Meats (lean)—Allow 2 or more 3-ounce servings daily—beef, fish, or chicken

Milk or milk products, preferably low fat—2 cups

Cereals, breads (whole grain or enriched), potatoes, or rice—4 or more servings daily (1 serv-

NUTRITIONAL NEED CHART

DID YOU CONSUME:

a. 6 or more ozs. of meat, including beef, fish, and chicken?
b. 2 cups of milk or milk products?
c. * 4 or more servings of bread or cereals? (1 serving is 1 slice of bread, or ¾ cup dry ready-to-eat cereal, or ½ cup cooked cereal)
d. 4 or more servings of vegetables and fruits?
e. * 2 tablespoons of fats or oils?

ing is 1 slice of bread, or ¾ cup of ready-to-eat cereal, or ½ cup cooked cereal). (This may be reduced to less than 4 servings if you are on a weight loss diet.)

Fruits and vegetables—4 or more servings

Fats or oils, preferably polyunsaturated—2 tablespoons (This may be reduced to less than 2 tablespoons if you are on a weight loss diet.)

Fill in the table on the page below by referring to column 2 on your Eating Behavior Charts, and learn whether you are eating a nutritionally balanced diet.

* A weight loss diet may require less of these items.

DAY 1	DAY 2	DAY 3	DAY 4	DAY 5	DAY 6	DAY 7

If on any day you omitted foods in groups a, b, c, d, or e, or ate less than the indicated amounts— your nutritional needs were not being met.

---

3. Are You Eating Too Much?

Your body requires a certain amount of food as fuel to make it operate each day. If your weight is stable, the amount you take in is used up to provide energy for your body.

Therefore, your weight is a function of:

1. The energy value of food eaten
2. The energy expended in the course of your daily activities

To meet the average daily nutritional requirements, you only need about 1200 to 1400 calories each day. If you wish to lose weight, you must reduce your intake until it is closer to this minimal daily nutritional requirement.

There are individuals who, because of their body size and physical activity, may require fewer than 1200 calories to lose weight and others who may lose weight on 1600 calories or more.

TASK NO. 4 (Optional)

Work the following problem:
From the calorie column on the charts, record here the average number of calories consumed per day.

Day 1 _____

Day 2 _____

Day 3 _____

Day 4 _____

Day 5 _____

Day 6 _____

Day 7 _____

Total calories: _____

Now divide 7 into the total calories

_____

The average calories consumed per day
equals _____

Subtract 1200 from this average:

_____

This figure is the number of calories you
consume each day greater than that required to meet your minimal nutritional
needs.

4. Where Does Your Eating Take Place?

The specific location at which eating takes place
becomes a cue to food consumption. To reduce
food intake, it is important to reduce the number
of cues to eating.

TASK NO. 5

Refer to column 4 of the Eating Behavior Charts and answer the following questions:

1. Do you eat at a specific place in your home?
   yes _____ no _____
2. Indicate the location by circling one or more of the following:
   a. Kitchen
   b. Dining room
   c. Family room
   d. Den
   e. Bedroom
   f. Living room
   g. _____
   h. _____
3. Indicate the location of your eating away from home by circling one of the following:
   a. Snack bar
   b. Office desk
   c. Car
   d. Neighbor's house
   e. _____
   f. _____

5. What Activities or Distractions Cause You to Overeat?

Most people do not realize the number of different situations that contribute to their overeating. Eating becomes associated with these situations and, as a result, is often stimulated by them rather than by hunger.

TASK NO. 6

Refer to column 5 on the Eating Behavior Charts and circle those situations that frequently contribute to your overeating.

Add any other situations that are associated with your overeating.

Situations at home
1. Clearing table
2. Eating off others' plates
3. Preparing foods
4. Entertaining a neighbor
5. Watching TV
6. 3 o'clock milk and cookies with children returning home from school
7. _____
8. _____

Situations away from home
1. Coffee break at office
2. Parties
3. Restaurants
4. Movies
5. Shopping
6. _____
7. _____
8. _____

Refer to column 5 on the Eating Behavior Charts to determine what distractions occur while you are eating.

These distractions cause you to be unaware of the amount of food you eat, and keep you from appreciating its taste.

You may discover that much of your eating is automatic. In fact, you may eat while engaging in these activities even though you are not hungry.

TASK NO. 7

Circle below the activities that occurred while you were eating.

1. Watching TV
2. Reading
3. Listening to stereo or radio
4. Knitting/sewing
5. _____
6. _____
7. _____
8. _____

6. What Feelings Cause You to Overeat?

Review column 6 on the Eating Behavior Charts and determine here what emotional feelings were frequently associated with your eating.

TASK NO. 8

Circle the emotional feelings that frequently occurred in conjunction with your eating.

1. Anger _____
2. Anxiety _____
3. Sadness or loneliness _____
4. Tiredness _____
5. _____
6. _____

7. Evaluating the Effect of Other Persons on Your Eating Behavior

Now refer to column 7 on the Eating Behavior Charts to determine the influence of the persons around you on your eating behavior. Give some thought to whether these people make positive, negative, or neutral comments about your eating behavior.

TASK NO. 9

In the chart below, indicate (+) for positive comments, (−) for negative comments, and (0) for neutral comments about your eating behavior for each person whose name you will enter in the appropriate place.

COMMENTS BY PERSONS AROUND YOU:

1. *Nagging*
2. *Praising your efforts to diet*
3. *Making fun of your efforts to diet*
4. *Commenting on your motivation and determination*
5. *Complimenting you on your present obese state*
6. *Showing pleasure at anticipating the new you*
7. *Reminding you of your previous failures*
8. *Inviting you to eat fattening foods*
9. *Inviting you to watch while they eat fattening foods*
10. *Telling you not to discuss your dieting*
11. *Making derogratory comments about your overweight*

Name of person	Name of person	Name of person	Name of person	Name of person	Name of person
——	——	——	——	——	——
——	——	——	——	——	——
——	——	——	——	——	——
——	——	——	——	——	——
——	——	——	——	——	——
——	——	——	——	——	——
——	——	——	——	——	——
——	——	——	——	——	——
——	——	——	——	——	——
——	——	——	——	——	——
——	——	——	——	——	——

8. Other Influences on Your Eating Behavior

What else have you learned from the Eating Behavior Charts concerning your specific eating problems?

Are there other factors that have a negative influence on your eating habits?

Look closely at your Eating Behavior Charts and see if you can determine other patterns that contribute to your specific problems.

TASK NO. 10

Record below any other observations concerning your eating behavior that you have noted from the Charts.

In this section you might give some attention to the specific times of day or night when your overeating occurs. You may have found that a specific meal once a week, or a number of times each week, causes you the most difficulty.

1. _____

2. _____

3. _____

4. _____

5. _____

6. _____

Those _____ on Your Eating

PART II

How to Change
Your Eating Behavior
and
Be on Your Way
to Permanent
Weight Loss

3.

Overcoming Your Specific Eating Problems

You have looked at your current eating behavior and determined your problem areas. Now you will focus on your specific problems and discover how to overcome them. The precise instructions in this section will then make it surprisingly easy for you to learn new eating patterns.

---

1. You Eat Too Fast—Slow Down!

Overweight people eat too fast. There is a time lag for signals traveling from the stomach to the brain, notifying it that sufficient food has arrived.

Therefore, if you eat quickly, your hunger won't be satisfied until after your stomach has received more food than you need. By increasing your eating time—that is, eating more slowly—you will find it easier to eat less. In addition, you will have greater appreciation and enjoyment of your food.

You must make a deliberate effort to eat slowly. Here are a number of techniques you can use:

1. Do not pick up a second morsel of food until you have completely chewed and swallowed the first one.
2. Take a rest period after a certain number of mouthfuls.
3. Put your fork down frequently.
4. Pay more attention to the taste, smell, and texture of the food.
5. Try to be the last person to finish each course of a meal.

Until now, you have probably been a gulper and have never really enjoyed or appreciated your food. From now on, eat each meal in no less than twenty to thirty minutes. Develop a definite *rhythm* to your eating. Approach each meal from the standpoint of *"how am I going to pace myself?"* This is a crucial step you must take to successfully lose weight and maintain the weight loss.

Do the following exercise:

1. Select a small food item of your choice, such as a piece of bread or a cookie.

2. Try to eat this item in no less than ten minutes.

3. Pace yourself in regard to the frequency of your bites.

4. Take small bites and completely chew and swallow each before taking another.

---

2. You Eat Too Much—Here Is Your Slow-Up to Slim-Down Diet

This diet emphasizes foods that help bring about the desired new eating behavior. It does this by enabling you to get greater satisfaction from the foods you eat.

The two basic categories of foods that will help you to practice your new eating behavior are the *slow-up liquids* and the *slow-up solids*.

SLOW-UP LIQUIDS

1. You will eat less and be more satisfied after drinking a liquid. Therefore, begin each meal with a *slow-up liquid*.
2. Slow-up liquids have no calories, low calories, or negligible calories. Examples are:

   8-ounces water
   8-ounces vegetable or tomato juice
   8-ounces diet beverage

TASK NO. 12

Circle the slow-up liquids which appeal to you.

1. 8-ounces tomato juice
2. 8-ounces diet beverage
3. 8-ounces iced tea with artificial sweetener
4. 8-ounces club soda with lemon or lime juice for flavor
5. 8-ounces vegetable or meat broth

SLOW-UP SOLIDS

1. You will eat less and be more satisfied by eating foods which take longer to eat.
2. Each meal must contain at least one slow-up solid.
3. The three groups of slow-up solids are:
   a. Foods that have negligible calories, or so few calories that they can be eaten in unlimited quantity. Examples:
      1. Lettuce
      2. Celery
      3. Cauliflower
      4. Spinach
      5. Broccoli
      6. Asparagus
      7. Cucumbers
   b. Foods that provide a lot to eat and relatively few calories. Examples:
      1. Cantaloupe
      2. Grapefruit
      3. Strawberries
      4. Blueberries
      5. Apple
      6. Pineapple
   c. Foods that take longer to eat because they require more work in order to eat them. Examples:
      1. Fish (which has not been filleted)
      2. Crab in the hard shell
      3. Soft-boiled egg in the shell

TASK NO. 13

Circle below the negligible calorie slow-up solids which appeal to you.

1. Cauliflower
2. Lettuce
3. Celery
4. Spinach
5. Broccoli
6. Asparagus
7. Kale
8. Brussel sprouts
9. Eggplant
10. Mushrooms
11. Cucumbers
12. Okra
13. Peppers
14. Radishes
15. Rhubarb
16. Sauerkraut
17. Watercress
18. Turnip greens
19. Cabbage
20. Collards
21. Mustard greens
22. Summer squash
23. Endive
24. Beet greens
25. Dandelion greens

Another factor that will increase your eating satisfaction is to enhance the presentation of the food. This can be accomplished by:

1. Completely filling your plate.
    a. Use a smaller-sized plate, or
    b. Completely spread the food over the plate, or
    c. Add negligible calorie foods to the plate.
2. Use of decorative items such as parsley, watercress, chicory, lettuce, and carrots.

SNACKING FOR GREATER SATISFACTION

It is helpful to have a number of snack periods each day (mid-morning, mid-afternoon, and mid-evening).

Rules for Snacking:

1. Each snack period must start with a slow-up liquid.
2. The slow-up liquid may be followed by low or negligible calorie slow-up solids.
3. You may include any food item not eaten at the preceding meal.

Here Is Your Slow-Up to Slim-Down Menu Model

BREAKFAST

Slow-Up Liquid • tomato juice, 8 ounces

Slow-Up Solid • 1 egg (soft-boiled in shell), or egg omelet with mushroom, spinach, or onions

1 slice bread
1 pat margarine

or

Slow-Up Solid • cold cereal with strawberries or blueberries, ¾ cup

1 cup skim milk

LUNCH

Slow-Up Liquid • tomato juice or iced tea, 8 ounces

fish, chicken, or lean meat, 3 ounces

2 slices of bread
1 pat margarine

vegetable, ½ cup

Slow-Up Solid • cantaloupe or grapefruit, unsectioned

DINNER

Slow-Up Liquid • club soda with lime or lemon wedge, or tomato juice, 8 ounces

fish, chicken, or lean meat, 3 ounces

2 vegetables (1 cup)

1 cup skim milk

Slow-Up Solid • salad of lettuce and sliced cucumbers

• ½ cup blueberries

Completely familiarize yourself with your Slow-Up to Slim-Down menu model so that each day you can select and visualize the food items you plan to eat at each meal or snack time.

During the day, be continually aware of those foods you have eaten and those which you will eat later in the day.

TASK NO. 14

1. Fill in your menu model for:

Breakfast

Lunch

Dinner

2. Choose those food items which appeal to you and approximate most closely the food items you usually eat.

3. Visualize these food items and think about them until you can readily recall them to mind.

SEVEN-DAY SLOW-UP TO SLIM-DOWN TRAINING PROGRAM

The sample menus on pages 65–74 will help you practice the slow-up method for weight loss, and you should follow them faithfully during the seven-day training program. Let the meals guide you to a new and more constructive approach to your eating.

Women may use the menu models as they are presented. Men may use the same models by adding approximately 400 calories daily. This can be done conveniently by use of the chart below or by referring to any calorie counter.

BEVERAGES	*80 calories*
Beer or carbonated beverages	6 ounces
Hard liquor	1 ounce
Red wines	2 ounces
White wines	3 ounces

BREAD (carbohydrate)	*70 calories*
White, whole wheat, rye	1 slice
English muffin	½
Saltine crackers	5
Dry cereal	¾ cup
Cooked cereal	½ cup
Spaghetti or macaroni	½ cup
Potato	1 small

FRUITS	*40 calories*
Apple	1 small
Apple juice or sauce	½ cup
Banana	½ small
Blackberries, raspberries strawberries, blueberries	⅔ cup
Cantaloupe	¼
Cherries	10 large
Grapefruit	½
Grapefruit juice	½ cup
Honeydew	⅛ medium
Orange	1 small
Orange juice	½ cup
Peach	1 medium
Pear	1 small
Pineapple	½ cup

Pineapple juice	½ cup
Plums	2 medium
Tomato	1 large
Watermelon	1 cup

MEAT (fish or poultry products)   *75 calories*

Lean meat and poultry	1 ounce
Egg	1
Fish: flounder, haddock, halibut	1 ounce
salmon, tuna, crab, lobster	¼ cup
shrimp, clams, oysters	5 small

MILK PRODUCTS   *80 calories*

Whole milk	½ cup
Buttermilk (from skim milk)	1 cup
Skim milk (1%)	1 cup
2% milk	¾ cup
Cottage cheese (plain)	½ cup
Cottage cheese (creamed)	⅓ cup
Cheese, hard (i.e., cheddar)	1 ounce

VEGETABLES   *40 calories*

Artichokes	Peas, green	½ cup
Beets	Pumpkin	serving
Carrots	Turnip	for each
Onions	Squash, winter	vegetable

Notice that in each meal on the following menu models, the slow-up liquids and slow-up solids are indicated by a heavy dot (•).

Slow-up liquids for breakfast may include: hot coffee, hot tea, iced coffee, iced tea, or tomato juice; for lunch: cold or hot tomato juice, bouillon, clear broth (fat removed), coffee, tea, low calorie soda, or low calorie lemonade; for dinner: Bloody

Mary mix (low calorie) on ice with lemon (no liquor), Club Soda with wedge of lime, lemon, or orange, low calorie soda, hot or cold tomato juice, or bouillon.

— Monday —

BREAKFAST . . . .

- Hot coffee, hot tea, iced coffee, or iced tea, 8 ounces

- ½ grapefruit

1 poached egg on toast

1 pat margarine

1 cup skim milk

LUNCH . . . .

- Cold or hot tomato juice, bouillon, clear broth (fat removed), coffee, tea, or lemonade, 8 ounces

Open-faced sandwich of 3 ounces tuna fish on 1 slice bread

- Unsweetened dill pickle, radishes, 2 slices of tomato, lettuce, mayonnaise (2 teaspoons)

DINNER . . . .

- Bloody Mary mix (low calorie) on ice with lemon (no liquor), club soda with wedge of lime, lemon, or orange, low calorie soda, hot or cold tomato juice, or bouillon, 8 ounces

Soy-Sauce Chicken,* 4 ounces

½ cup cooked enriched rice

Asparagus served cold with lemon wedges

• **Tossed green salad with Slim-Down Diet Salad Dressing** *

• **Hot Cinnamon Apples** *

1 cup skim milk

Hot or cold coffee or tea

RECIPES

* Soy-Sauce Chicken—Remove skin from cut-up pieces of chicken. Place in oven roasting bag; sprinkle with soy sauce and garlic powder. Bake at 350° for 45 minutes or until done.

* Slim-Down Diet Salad Dressing—Mix together ½ cup tomato juice, 2 tablespoons wine vinegar or lemon juice, 1 tablespoon onion, chopped, 2 to 3 drops olive oil.

* Hot Cinnamon Apples—Slice a fresh apple and place on a sheet of aluminum foil. Sprinkle with orange juice, cinnamon, and low calorie sweetener. Bake at 350° for 30 minutes or until done.

— Tuesday —

BREAKFAST . . . .

• Hot coffee, hot tea, iced coffee, or iced tea, 8 ounces

• ½ cup blueberries or

• 1 cup strawberries

¾ cup dry cereal

1 cup skim milk

LUNCH . . . .

- Cold or hot tomato juice, bouillon, clear broth (fat removed), coffee, tea, or lemonade, 8 ounces

Chicken salad, 3 ounces, with 2 teaspoons mayonnaise and lemon juice

- ½ head lettuce, shredded with radishes, spring onions, celery, capers, shredded purple cabbage

Use Slim-Down Diet Salad Dressing (p. 65)

1 slice of bread
1 pat margarine

1 cup skim milk

DINNER . . . .

- Bloody Mary mix (low calorie) on ice with lemon (no liquor), club soda with wedge of lime, lemon, or orange, low calorie soda, hot or cold tomato juice, or bouillon, 8 ounces

Beef-Ka-Bob,* 3 ounces

1 small baked potato
1 pat margarine

Brussel sprouts served hot with lemon wedge

- Tossed green salad with Slim-Down Diet Salad Dressing

- ½ grapefruit served cold or hot, and topped with a strawberry

RECIPES

* Beef-Ka-Bob—Place beef chunks on skewer with cherry tomatoes, onion, and green pepper. Sprinkle with salt and pepper. Broil.

— Wednesday —

BREAKFAST . . . .

- Hot coffee, hot tea, iced coffee, or iced tea, 8 ounces

½ cup unsweetened orange juice

- Cinnamon French Toast *

LUNCH . . . .

- Cold or hot tomato juice, bouillon, clear broth (fat removed), coffee, tea, or lemonade, 8 ounces

open-faced, grilled sandwich of 1 ounce shredded hard cheese with slices of tomato and sprinkled with oregano on one slice bread

- sweet and sour cucumber slices marinated in wine vinegar, 2 teaspoons oil, and low calorie sweetener, with chopped fresh scallions (drain before serving)

1 fresh peach

1 cup skim milk

DINNER . . . .

- Bloody Mary mix (low calorie) or ice with lemon (no liquor), club soda with wedge of lime, lemon, or orange, low calorie soda, hot or cold tomato juice, or bouillon, 8 ounces

Baked Fish Creole,* 3 ounces

½ cup lima beans, topped with 1 pat margarine

- Baked Acorn Squash,* ½ cup

1 cup skim milk

Baked apple with 1 teaspoon sugar

68

* *Cinnamon French Toast*—Mix 1 egg together with ¼ cup skim milk, vanilla, and cinnamon. Soak 2 slices of bread in mixture and fry with 1 teaspoon margarine. Top with berries.

* *Baked Fish Creole*—Put small amount of tomato juice on bottom of casserole dish. Layer fish fillets with thinly sliced onion and green pepper. Top with more tomato juice, crushed garlic clove, salt, and pepper. Bake at 350° for 20 minutes or until fish flakes easily when tested with a fork.

* *Baked Acorn Squash*—Quarter a raw squash. Place in baking pan. Pour 1 tablespoon orange juice on each quarter. Sprinkle with cinnamon and low calorie powdered sweetener. Cover with aluminum foil. Bake 1 hour at 350° or until squash is tender.

— Thursday —

BREAKFAST . . . .

- Hot coffee, hot tea, iced coffee, or iced tea, 8 ounces

½ cup unsweetened grapefruit juice

- ¼ cup cottage cheese on slice of toast, cut in quarters

1 cup skim milk

LUNCH . . . .

- Cold or hot tomato juice, bouillon, clear broth (fat removed), coffee, tea, or lemonade, 8 ounces

Cold fish salad, 3 ounces fish

- ½ head of lettuce, shredded, with radishes, spring onions, celery, capers, and tomato

dressing—oil (1 tablespoon) and vinegar

1 slice bread

1 cup skim milk

DINNER . . . .

- Bloody Mary mix (low calorie) on ice with lemon (no liquor), club soda with wedge of lime, lemon, or orange, low calorie soda, hot or cold tomato juice, or bouillon, 8 ounces

Chicken Tetrazzini,* 3 ounces, served on ½ cup cooked noodles

Marinated Stringbeans,* ½ cup
Plate of sliced cucumbers and pimiento on ice

- Pineapple boat (¼ medium fresh pineapple sliced thinly and served in shell)

RECIPES

* Chicken Tetrazzini—Remove skin from chicken. Steam chicken. Remove chicken from pot. Skim off fat from surface of the broth. In a small amount of fat-free broth, cook mushrooms, sliced celery, and green pepper. Add salt and pepper to broth. Slice chicken from the bone and add to the vegetable/broth mixture. With the one-half cup cooked wide noodles, make a bed and pour the chicken/vegetable mixture on top.

* Marinated Stringbeans—Cook frozen stringbeans for five minutes, allowing them to remain crisp. Drain and cool. In a separate bowl, mix 1 teaspoon vegetable oil, ¼ teaspoon dry mustard, salt and pepper to taste, and 3 tablespoons wine vinegar. Pour this mixture over the green beans and refrigerate for 2 hours. Drain stringbeans before serving.

— Friday —

BREAKFAST . . . .

- Hot coffee, hot tea, iced coffee, or iced tea, 8 ounces
- 1 fresh orange, sliced

½ cup hot cereal

1 cup skim milk

Slice of toast
1 pat of margarine

LUNCH . . . .

• Cold or hot tomato juice, bouillon, clear broth (fat removed), coffee, tea, or lemonade, 8 ounces

Sandwich of smoked salmon, 3 ounces, with 1 ounce farmer cheese, and capers on two slices bread

1 cup skim milk

• Bed of lettuce, sliced tomato, celery and carrot sticks

DINNER . . . .

• Bloody Mary mix (low calorie) on ice with lemon (no liquor), club soda with wedge of lime, lemon, or orange, low calorie soda, hot or cold tomato juice, or bouillon, 8 ounces

Chinese Shrimp,* 4 ounces, served on a bed of ½ cup cooked enriched rice

• Salad of shredded lettuce, sliced radishes, and tomato

Baked Whole Fresh Pear *

RECIPES

* Chinese Shrimp—Heat 6 tablespoons of fat-free broth in a heavy skillet. Toss in 2 ounces of fresh or canned bean sprouts, sliced onions, sliced green pepper, and celery (or Chinese celery if available). Cook this mixture on a high heat, tossing constantly for 2 to 3 minutes. Add 4 ounces of cooked shrimp and toss until heated. Serve over cooked rice.

Baked Pears—Remove skins from fresh pears. Place in baking dish. Pour orange juice over pears till bottom of pan is covered with juice. Sprinkle cinnamon and low calorie powdered sweetener over pears. Cover with aluminum foil. Bake at 350° for 60 minutes. (Use only 1 teaspoon of remaining syrup over serving).

— Saturday —

BREAKFAST . . . .

- Hot coffee, hot tea, iced coffee, or iced tea, 8 ounces

1 ounce hard cheese, shredded and broiled on top of 1 slice toast, quartered

1 cup skim milk

- Baked apple with 1 teaspoon sugar

LUNCH . . . .

- Cold or hot tomato juice, bouillon, clear broth (fat removed), coffee, tea, or lemonade, 8 ounces

- Greek salad (diced tomatoes, cucumbers, green peppers, sliced sweet onion, and 1 ounce feta cheese)

Dressing of oil (1 tablespoon), vinegar, and oregano

2 slices of toast
2 pats of margarine

DINNER . . . .

- Bloody Mary mix (low calorie) on ice with lemon (no liquor), club soda with wedge of lime, lemon, or orange, low calorie soda, hot or cold tomato juice, or bouillon, 8 ounces

Garlic veal (broiled veal chop with minced garlic),
4 ounces

Ratatouille *

1 cup skim milk

• Tossed green salad of parsley and sliced celery
with Slim-Down Diet Salad Dressing

Hot Banana and Pineapple Compote *

RECIPES

* Ratatouille—*(This can be made ahead and stored in the
refrigerator.) Dice 1 small eggplant, 2 small zucchini squash,
1 large onion, and 1 green pepper. Add a can of whole
tomatoes or 2 fresh tomatoes. Add 2 minced cloves of
garlic, salt and pepper. Cook on top of stove for 3 to 4 hours.
(Cover until mixture comes to a boil; then uncover and let
simmer until liquid evaporates.) Serve hot or cold. Serves
5 or 6.*

* Hot Banana and Pineapple Compote—*Slice ½ banana and
6 pineapple cubes. Put in aluminum foil. Add 2 teaspoons
pineapple juice, cinnamon, and low calorie powdered sweetener. Close aluminum foil and bake for 15 minutes at 350
degrees. (Use pineapple packed in its own juice.)*

— Sunday —

BREAKFAST . . . .

• Hot coffee, hot tea, iced coffee, or iced tea,
8 ounces

• ½ grapefruit (unsectioned)

1 egg omelet with filling composed of 1 or more of
the following vegetables: cooked spinach, mushrooms, onions, chives, or green pepper

1 cup skim milk

1 slice toast
1 pat margarine

LUNCH . . . .

- Cold or hot tomato juice, bouillon, clear broth (fat removed), coffee, tea, or lemonade, 8 ounces

- Open-faced sandwich of sliced chicken, 3 ounces, with sliced tomato, lettuce, and mayonnaise (1 teaspoon) on one slice bread

1 cup skim milk

Unsweetened dill pickles

DINNER . . . .

- Bloody Mary mix (low calorie) on ice with lemon (no liquor), club soda with wedge of lime, lemon, or orange, low calorie soda, hot or cold tomato juice, or bouillon, 8 ounces

Cabbage Rolls,* 4 ounces of meat, and ½ cup cooked enriched rice

½ cup peas and mushrooms

Oranged Carrots,* ½ cup

Fruit cup (2 slices canned pineapple in its own juice with ½ cup mandarin orange sections)

RECIPES

Cabbage Rolls—Mix 4 ounces extra lean meat with ½ cup cooked rice. Parboil 1 head of cabbage so that the leaves can be separated. To meat/rice mixture add garlic powder, salt, and pepper. Put 1 tablespoon of meat mixture into a single cabbage leaf; fold like a pocket. Arrange these cabbage rolls in a casserole dish. Layer alternately with sliced onions and extra cabbage leaves, and remaining cabbage rolls. Add lemon juice and low carorie sweetener to taste, to tomato juice, and pour over the casserole. Cover and simmer for 1 hour. Before serving, place casserole (if in an oven-proof dish) under the broiler for a minute to brown.

Oranged Carrots—Shred fresh carrots. Cook with fresh or frozen orange juice. Add low calorie sweetener.

EXERCISE IS IMPORTANT

In addition to your Slow-Up to Slim-Down Diet, another way to lose weight is to increase your daily exercise. You can help your weight loss efforts by expending more energy than found in the food you eat. Many people have found that they have less appetite and therefore consume less food after exercising.

TASK NO. 15

Circle below those activities you engage in on a regular basis.

Indicate below how many minutes per week you spend in each activity.

1. Walking up stairs _____
2. Making beds _____
3. Washing dishes _____
4. Scrubbing floors _____
5. Yard work _____
6. Tennis _____
7. Golf _____
8. Jogging _____
9. Volley ball _____
10. Baseball _____
11. Swimming _____
12. Others _____ _____
13. _____ _____

The following chart will give you some idea of how many minutes you must engage in various activities to burn up the calories contained in some common foods. By using the chart, you will better understand the part

EXERCISE REQUIRED TO BURN UP CALORIES OF VARIOUS FOODS

FOOD	Calories	Jogging or Swimming
½ cup cauliflower	11	1
1 2-inch-round cracker	15	2
½ cup strawberries	25	3
½ grapefruit	40	4
1 slice bread	70	7
1 egg	80	8
1½ ounces (1 slice) pound cake	170	17
3 ounces ground beef	210	21
1 slice blueberry pie, 5½ ounces (1/6 of 9-inch pie)	380	38

For example, in order to burn up the 11 calories in ½ cup of cauliflower, you would need to jog for one minute, or play tennis for two minutes, or walk up stairs for one minute.

that exercise currently plays in using up calories for you, and how an increase in exercise can make a difference in your weight loss program.

Now is the time to resume a particular sport or physical activity that interested you in the past.

MINUTES OF ACTIVITY

Tennis	Walking Up Stairs	Washing Dishes	Making Beds	Sitting, Relaxed
2	1	4	2	11
2	1	5	2	15
3	2	8	3	23
6	2	13	6	40
10	4	23	10	70
12	5	26	12	80
24	10	56	24	170
30	12	69	30	210
54	21	126	54	380

BEFORE UNDERTAKING ANY SIGNIFICANT INCREASE IN YOUR LEVEL OF PHYSICAL ACTIVITY, CONSULT YOUR PHYSICIAN.

Now you are ready to start your Slow-Up to Slim-Down Diet.

Begin a period of seven days during which you will strictly adhere to the week's menu models on pages 65–74. At the end of this trial, weigh yourself once more. If you have lost 1 to 3 pounds, you are doing fine; continue practicing your new eating behavior.

If you lose more than 3 pounds, you are losing weight too rapidly. It takes time to learn new eating behavior and a too rapid weight loss will not enable you to convert your newly practiced patterns to firmly established habits. Therefore, during the second week, you must consume food containing 500 calories more each day. In planning your daily menu, consult a calorie chart and distribute the extra 500 calories per day in whatever manner you please. If the extra 500 calories per day result in no weight loss during the second week, resume your original menu plan.

If you have not lost any weight after your first week on the diet, keep an accurate record of your food intake for seven more days to see if you depart from the menu models. If you find that you strictly adhered to the menu models and still did not lose 1 to 3 pounds after the second week, consult your doctor for a further reduction in your food intake.

It is important that you weigh yourself once each week. You should weigh yourself at the same time of day, preferably upon arising in the morning.

3. You Eat in Too Many Places— Limit Locations

If you eat in many different places in your home, it is essential that you discontinue this behavior.

Select one place where you will eat all your meals—either the dining room or the kitchen. Eat at a specific seat in this room and do not vary this position.

Remember, to limit the number of cues which suggest eating, *you must limit the number of places connected with eating.*

Use a colorful place mat, china setting, glass, and cutlery set to remind you that this is your particular eating territory.

TASK NO. 16

1. Determine in which room you will eat. Locate your place at the table.

2. Eat all your food at this spot. Select a colorful place mat for your place setting.

4. Eliminate Activities and Distractions That Contribute to Overeating

As we have seen, eating often occurs along with other activities such as watching TV or reading. These activities then become cues to eating, even at times when you are not feeling hungry.

It is important to develop the habit of eating all your meals without distraction, even if you are eating alone.

Concentrate on your food, and eating will become a more enjoyable experience which will more quickly lead to feelings of satiation.

TASK NO. 17

Review the activities that serve as distractions to your eating.

Refer to Task No. 6 and list these distractions below.

1. _____

2. _____

3. _____

4. _____

5. Emotions That Contribute to Your Overeating

Earlier you determined which feelings contributed to your overeating. Now you must learn how to deal with these feelings without overeating.

TASK NO. 18

Refer to Task No. 8 and record at this point those feelings that you most frequently found to be associated with your overeating.

_____

_____

_____

_____

HANDLING EMOTIONS THAT CAUSE YOU TO OVEREAT

There are two basic techniques you can use:
1. Express the feeling
   a. Verbally
   b. Physically

2. Divert your attention away from the feeling toward a pleasurable or relaxing activity or thought.

Here are some examples of how to apply these techniques for specific feelings:

ANGER

WHEN YOU ARE ANGRY, INSTEAD OF OVER-EATING:
1. Express the feeling to the person toward whom you are angry.
2. Talk about your anger to a person who will be supportive.
3. *Think* about expressing the anger directly toward the person who engendered it.
4. Physically express the anger by hitting a pillow or by engaging in some other physical activity.
5. Divert your attention from anger to a pleasurable thought.
6. Divert your attention by engaging in a pleasurable activity.

ANXIETY

WHEN YOU ARE ANXIOUS, INSTEAD OF OVER-EATING:
1. Use the muscular relaxation technique (page 110).
2. Engage in physical activity.

3. Divert your attention away from the anxious state by thinking about something pleasurable.
4. Engage in a pleasurable activity.
5. If the anxiety is caused by specific problems, talk to a supportive person and try to resolve the problems.

SADNESS AND LONELINESS

WHEN YOU ARE SAD, INSTEAD OF OVEREATING:
1. Talk to someone who is supportive.
2. Engage in a pleasurable activity.
3. Think about something pleasurable.
4. Find a substitute for food, such as companionship.

TIREDNESS

WHEN YOU ARE TIRED, INSTEAD OF OVEREATING:
1. Take a relaxing shower or bath.
2. Find a companion.
3. Begin to catch up on your needed sleep.

6. The People Around You—Are They Helping or Hurting Your Attempts to Lose Weight?

Earlier you concentrated on *situations* that contributed to your overeating. Now think about the *people* who affect your weight loss efforts.

Refer to Task no. 9 and note that some of the important people in your life are helpful, some are neutral, and others actually discourage your efforts at weight loss.

TASK NO. 19

Below write the names of the people in your environment who you feel are discouraging you in your efforts to lose weight.

Refer to Task no. 9 for this information.

1. _____

2. _____

3. _____

4. _____

5. _____

HOW TO DEAL WITH PEOPLE
WHO EXERT NEGATIVE INFLUENCES
ON YOUR EATING BEHAVIOR

1. Try asking everyone who makes negative comments about your eating behavior to cooperate in your efforts to lose weight.
2. Suggest that they try to make only positive remarks regarding your efforts.
3. You do not have to listen to them or engage in arguments with them.

If the above suggestions don't work, try some of the following techniques:

1. When the conversation becomes disturbing, change the subject to one of particular interest to the person you are talking with. This will divert his attention from the negative comments about your eating behavior.
2. Think of something pleasant or relaxing.

HOW YOU CAN RECEIVE EVEN GREATER ASSISTANCE FROM THOSE PERSONS IN YOUR ENVIRONMENT WHO ARE HELPFUL

After referring to Task no. 9, reward the positive behavior of the people who help your weight loss efforts by thanking them for their encouragement. Give them other suggestions so they can continue to help you. For example:

1. Ask them not to offer food to you.
2. Ask them not to eat fattening foods in your presence.
3. Ask them not to compliment you on your present over-weight appearance.
4. Ask them to comment only on your positive eating behavior.
5. Ask them to comment on the emerging new you and express their approval of that image.
6. Ask their assistance in deciding on rewards for your efforts.
7. Ask them if they are also interested in weight loss; they can be of enormous help by making it a mutual effort.
8. Ask for encouragement when you are having difficulty and your motivation needs a boost.

TASK NO. 20

List below the people who usually make encouraging remarks about your weight loss efforts.

1. _____

2. _____

3. _____

4. _____

5. _____

7. How to Deal with Other Problems— Coping with Specific Situations That Contribute to Your Overeating

1. If overeating occurs at restaurants or parties:
   a. Determine the low calorie foods that are available.
   b. Decide what and how much food fits your menu model.
   c. Eat slowly.

2. If overeating occurs at movies, ball games, or similar activities:
   a. Save food from your menu model for such occasions.
   b. Pace your eating.
   c. Take low calorie foods with you.

3. If overeating occurs as a result of having to serve food to guests:
   a. Do not feel obligated to eat the foods you serve to your guests.
   b. Serve yourself low calorie foods and drinks; your guests may also prefer these foods.
4. If overeating occurs during your coffee break:
   a. Send someone else for coffee.
   b. Go yourself only if food is not available.
   c. Take a thermos to work.
5. If you overeat when you pass the candy counter in drug stores or newspaper stands:
   a. Only buy items from a previously prepared list.
   b. Go to these places only after you have eaten.
   c. Take a low calorie food with you.
6. If overeating occurs while preparing meals:
   a. Drink water or noncaloric beverages.
   b. Eat only celery, carrots, or other low calorie foods.
   c. If possible, prepare food when you are not hungry; i.e., immediately after lunch, prepare dinner.
   d. Do not prepare fattening foods (particularly foods you cannot resist) for other members of the family. They can prepare these foods for themselves or get them away from home.

COPING WITH THE BINGE

If you find that you go on eating binges at particular times, plan to do something else at those times. For example, you might schedule a particular diversion, such as reading or doing crossword puzzles. You must switch to this specific activity at the time you usually find yourself tempted to overeat.

If you find that you binge because of the presence of certain foods, eliminate them from your house.

TASK NO. 21

Diverting your attention to a specific activity will help you avoid binging.

List below activities that can be readily available for this purpose (books, magazines, crossword puzzles, etc.).

1. _____

2. _____

3. _____

4. _____

COPING WITH THE SNACK

Plan to save foods from your menu model for snacks. During snack time, pace yourself so your eating can last longer. You may find it helpful to carry low calorie foods with you for these occasions.

Again, if you find certain foods are irresistible,

be sure that they are not available.

If there are specific times when you compulsively snack, think of interesting activities to divert your attention.

Remember the rules for snacking (see page 59).

TASK NO. 22

Certain foods have negligible calories and can be consumed as desired. Circle below those foods that appeal to you.

1. Coffee
2. Tea
3. Gelatin
4. Broth/bouillon
5. Lime juice/lemon juice
6. Unsweetened pickles
7. Raw vegetables—celery, cucumber, cauliflower

PART III

Practicing Your New
Eating Behavior
Can Be
Fun and Rewarding

4.

How to Reward Yourself

A behavior that is consistently followed by a reward tends to be repeated. Therefore, you must reward your new and desired eating behavior frequently.

THOUGHT REWARDS

Each time you use your new and constructive eating behavior, mentally associate that behavior with a pleasant image of yourself as a thin person. You will be giving up your old behavior, which was associated with a distressing image of yourself as a fat person.

**OLD EATING
BEHAVIOR
associated with the
FAT YOU**

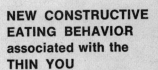

**NEW CONSTRUCTIVE
EATING BEHAVIOR
associated with the
THIN YOU**

For example, you are about to reach for a bag of potato chips as you watch TV. Immediately think of the *fat you,* which gives you a feeling of distress, and then push aside the bag of potato chips and associate this positive behavior with the image of the *thin you*—the person you would like to become. Accomplishing this will immediately give you pleasant feelings and will ultimately lead to a sense of control, pride, and self-mastery.

In summary, the positive and new eating behavior is immediately rewarded by pleasant feelings. When this pattern is repeated often enough, you will more automatically avoid those eating behaviors which were associated with *the fat you.*

1. The Fat You

In order to achieve thought rewards you must have a clear understanding of your body image. Before you begin your weight loss efforts, you have a self-image that is dramatically colored by being overweight. We refer to this as the *fat you*.

The following material will help you look at yourself in a way that will demonstrate the various aspects of your self-image—your self-esteem, body image, appearance, and health.

YOUR SELF-ESTEEM—
HOW YOU FEEL ABOUT YOURSELF

Overweight causes you to have many negative feelings about yourself. You may find that you do not like yourself, that you feel inadequate, weak, dependent or helpless. You may even feel like a failure.

These feelings have little relationship to your actual abilities, but they are an enormous burden and may, in fact, lead to poor performance in many areas of your life.

Determine factors about your low self-esteem by circling those that apply to you. List any others.

1. You do not like yourself.
2. You feel inadequate.
3. You feel weak.
4. You feel like a failure.
5. You feel helpless.
6. Other feelings associated with your overweight:

_____

_____

_____

YOUR BODY IMAGE— HOW YOU FEEL ABOUT YOUR BODY

As a result of being overweight, you have a number of feelings about your own body which you do not like. They are not entirely related to the way your body actually is, but are strongly influenced by emotional discomfort about various parts of your body.

In many cases, you may actually see your body as much worse than it really is. By recognizing those parts of your body that dissatisfy you, you will be in a better position to improve the image of yourself through your weight loss efforts.

Take a look at yourself in the mirror. Try to be as objective as possible about your body, its shape, and dimensions.

Select from the list below, those parts of your body which you are not happy about and would like to change.

1. Face _____
2. Chin _____
3. Neck _____
4. Chest _____
5. Arms _____
6. Abdomen _____
7. Hips _____
8. Buttocks _____
9. Thighs _____
10. Legs _____
11. Feet _____
12. Other _____

YOUR APPEARANCE—
HOW YOU THINK OTHER PEOPLE SEE YOU

You may feel that you are physically unattractive to others—that your face, arms, legs, or other parts of your body are unattractive. You may even be ashamed to be seen in public.

The idea of wearing a bathing suit or a tennis outfit may terrify you. Or you may be disgusted with your inability to find clothing to hide the fat.

You may tend to avoid social situations because of your feelings of unattractiveness. You may actually believe that your family or friends are embarrassed to be seen with you.

TASK NO. 25

The following are concerns you may have regarding your overweight appearance. Circle those that apply and list any others.

1. Ashamed to be seen in public?

2. Feel disgusted when you look at yourself in the mirror?

3. Unable to find attractive clothing?

4. Unable to fit into your clothing?

5. Take a good look at yourself in the mirror. Look at yourself from all angles. Notice those aspects of yourself that you find most unattractive.

   List below the parts of your body that you feel are repulsive to you or to others.

   _____

   _____

6. Other aspects of your appearance (related to your being overweight) that concern you.

   _____

   _____

YOUR HEALTH—
THE PHYSICAL EFFECTS OF OVERWEIGHT

Your overweight condition may have some special health significance for you, either because of some problem you presently have or because of a family history of illness that is complicated by overweight.

TASK NO. 26

Complete the following items concerning the effect of overweight on your health:

1. Indicate here any health problems you are currently having.

_____

_____

2. List here any illnesses that run in your family which may be complicated by overweight.

_____

_____

_____

BEING OVERWEIGHT IS A HANDICAP IN CERTAIN SPORTS THAT YOU WOULD OTHERWISE ENJOY

Your weight may interfere with activities such as tennis, bowling, golf, swimming, or dancing. It may even be difficult for you to perform necessary physical activity such as walking or climbing stairs. Although you engage in some of these activities, you may find that you become fatigued too readily.

TASK NO. 27

The following are difficulties you may experience as the result of your over-weight: circle those that apply. List any others.

1. You have difficulty walking.

2. You have difficulty climbing stairs.

3. You tire easily.

4. You have difficulty engaging in the following athletic activities:
   a. tennis
   b. golf
   c. swimming
   d. bicycling
   e. football
   f. basketball
   g. baseball
   h. badminton
   i. volleyball
   j. _____

5. You have difficulty engaging in the following nonathletic activities:
   a. gardening

b. household chores
c. walking the dog
d. carrying the children
e. carrying the groceries
f. _____

6. You have difficulty engaging in the following job-related activities: List them.

   a. _____
   b. _____
   c. _____
   d. _____

7. List other activities that are impaired by your overweight.

_____

THE FAT YOU—
YOUR CURRENT SELF-ESTEEM

You have taken a good look at yourself by working through the material on the preceding pages. Now conjure up a realistic image of yourself related to your overweight condition. This realistic image is negative and displeasing to you. Thinking about it causes you to become uncomfortable.

Remember this discomfort, because it will be used as a means of helping you to shape new eating behaviors.

TASK NO. 28

Write in the highlights of your current self-esteem from the work you have done on the previous pages.

The Fat You

SELF-WORTH _____
_____
_____
_____

BODY IMAGE _____ _____
_____
_____
_____

APPEARANCE _____
_____
_____
_____

HEALTH AND ACTIVITIES _____
_____
_____
_____

THIS IS THE COMPOSITE OF THE **FAT YOU.**

2. The Thin You

When you become thin, you will view yourself in a more pleasing manner. Thoughts about this new image of yourself should be associated with a feeling of relaxation and sense of well-being which will serve as an incentive for practicing your new eating behaviors.

Look at what you would like to be in terms of the component parts of the thin you:

1. Increased self-esteem
2. More pleasing body image
3. More attractive appearance
4. Improved health and ability to engage in psysical activities

TASK NO. 29

Fill in the banks with the image you would like to have of yourself when you reach your desired weight. Choose from the examples and add others.

1. SELF-ESTEEM
   Feeling assertive, confident, elated, having sense of achievement,

   _____

   _____

2. BODY IMAGE
   Comfortable about parts of your body you considered unattractive (i.e., arms, legs, chin, abdomen),

   _____

   _____

3. APPEARANCE
   Attractive, popular, socially at ease,

   _____

   _____

4. HEALTH AND ACTIVITIES
Vigorous, energetic, free of health concerns, able to engage in tennis, swimming,

_____

_____

THIS IS THE COMPOSITE OF THE **THIN YOU.**

VISUALIZATION-RELAXATION TECHNIQUE

You are now ready to use the visualization-relaxation technique to help you lose weight. Remember, this is a method of getting an immediate reward for practicing your new eating patterns.

First you will think of yourself as _the fat you_ and this image will be associated with a feeling of distress.

TASK NO. 30
_____

1. Think of the composite _Fat You_ (in Task no. 28), in terms of the categories of diminished self-esteem, poor body image, unattractive appearance, and impaired health and declining activity tolerance—until you clearly see yourself in these dimensions.

2. Continue to think about the Fat You until you have a vivid visualization accompanied by a sense of *distress* and *anxiety*.

After you have visualized the composite *fat you* and have experienced a sense of discomfort, relax by visualizing a pleasant scene or experience. Recall a time and place when you felt comfortable and peaceful.

Associate this feeling of comfort and relaxation with the image of the composite *thin you.*

TASK NO. 31

1. Use your imagination to recall a very calm and peaceful scene that creates in your mind and body a sense of comfort and relaxation.
2. In such a scene, you may visualize yourself lying on a beach in the sun enjoying a fresh ocean breeze or in a mountain setting with comfortable cool air wafting past your face and body.
3. When you have thought about this situation until you are indeed comfortable and relaxed, associate that scene and the accompanying feeling with the composite Thin You, (including those features of self-esteem, good body image, pleasant

appearance, and increased sense of physical well-being which will become part of you when you reach your desired weight).

SUMMARY OF THE VISUALIZATION-RELAXATION TECHNIQUE

Tasks nos. 30 and 31 are used in the following manner: visualize the *fat you* until you experience anxiety.

Then, suddenly switch your thoughts to a calm and pleasant scene until you feel a sense of relaxation.

Then visualize the *thin you.*

TASK NO. 32

Do the following exercise ten times daily for one week:
1. Visualize the Fat You.
2. When you achieve feelings of anxiety, suddenly, SWITCH YOUR THOUGHTS, and now,
3. Think about a pleasant scene until you achieve a sense of relaxation.
4. When you are sufficiently relaxed, visualize the *Thin You.*

MUSCULAR RELAXATION CAN HELP

If thinking about a calm scene does not bring about a sense of relaxation, try muscular relaxation.

First tense various muscles and then suddenly release them. Doing this several times can help bring about generalized feelings of calm and relaxation.

TASK NO. 33

Below is an exercise to help you relax.

1. Clench your fists in order to tense the muscles of your hand. Notice the tension. Suddenly let your hands relax. Enjoy the relaxed and comfortable way they feel.

2. Next, tighten the muscles of your forearms and concentrate on the tension once again. Then let the muscles go limp and enjoy the sense of pleasant relaxation.

3. You can repeat this exercise with other large muscle groups, alternately tensing and then suddenly relaxing them. This feeling of muscular relaxation is what you are striving for in your attempts to reach a state of general relaxation.

APPLICATION OF VISUALIZATION-RELAXATION TECHNIQUE

When you are tempted to engage in an old eating behavior, such as reaching for a fattening food, relate this behavior to the composite *fat you.*

Visualize the fat, unhealthy, unattractive you until you experience a feeling of anxiety.

Refuse the fattening food, and be immediately rewarded by a feeling of calm and relaxation associated with the image of the *thin you.*

This serves as an immediate reward for constructive eating behavior and will help you to successfully avoid fattening foods.

TASK NO. 34

1. Think of a fattening food that you find particularly tempting.

   Write the name of the food here

   _____

2. Think of the composite image of the *Fat You.*

   When you sense a feeling of discomfort, imagine pushing the fattening food away from you.

3. SWITCH your thoughts to a picture of the *Thin You* associated with a feeling of relaxation.

3. Point Rewards

You have already practiced the visualization-relaxation technique which provided you with an immediate reward for practicing your new eating behaviors.

Now we will show you another method of immediate reward. You can assign points for practicing specific new eating behavior. Each time you practice a new eating behavior, give yourself a number of points. This assigning of points is a practical way of giving you an immediate reward for your new behavior, and can later be converted into a material reward.

On the next two pages you will find a list of new eating behaviors which you must practice. For each time you practice a new eating behavior, give yourself the suggested number of points.

THIS CHART SUMMARIZES THE EATING BEHAVIORS WHICH YOU MUST PRACTICE. LATER THE POINTS WILL BE CONVERTED TO REWARDS.

SUGGESTED POINTS

1. Eating each of the three main meals in no less than 20 to 30 minutes.

   2 points for each meal

2. Successfully avoiding temptation to binge.

   1 point for each success

3. Eating without distractions.

   1 point for each meal

4. Eating only at planned times (3 meals and snacks if they are included in *your* menu plan).

   1 point for each meal

5. Adhering rigidly to the menu model of your choice.

   1 point for each meal

6. Eating only at appropriate and designated places.

   1 point for each meal

7. Exercise. (Indicate number of minutes per day—)

   1 point per 5 minutes

8. Overcoming a specific situational eating problem, i.e.,
   a. Parties
   b. Restaurants
   c. Watching TV
   d. When neighbors visit
   e. When shopping (to drug store or supermarket)

   1 point suggested for each of the categories

f. Taking coffee break

g. Any special exposures to food stimuli (while preparing food for family or when clearing table) _____

1 point suggested for each of the categories

9. Not eating when the following emotional feelings occur.

a. Anger _____

b. Anxiety _____

c. Fatigue _____

d. Frustration _____

e. Sadness _____

f. Loneliness _____

g. Boredom _____

h. _____

i. _____

j. _____

1 point per success

10. *

* The remainder of the table can be tailored to your own specific problems.

TASK NO. 35

1. Circle on the chart above the eating behaviors which you must change.

2. Add all the points from the "Suggested Points" column that you can accumulate each day, if you practiced all your new eating behaviors. You can accumulate a maximum of _____ points each day.

3. Multiply the number of points possible per day by 7, to achieve the number of points you can accumulate each week.

You can accumulate a maximum of _____ points each week.

CONVERTING POINTS TO REWARDS

By using the chart below, you can choose rewards for practicing your new eating behavior. You may choose from these rewards, or substitute others which are more appropriate for you.

Total Points Per Week	Money	Gifts	Activities
40	$ 2.00	Lottery tickets	
60	$ 3.00		
80	$ 4.00		Movie
100	$ 5.00	Record	Get babysitter—take day off
200	$10.00	Hairdresser	
			Dinner out
300	$15.00	Clothes	
350	$20.00	Tennis Racket	

List below your personal choice of weekly rewards.

After each reward, indicate the number of points that will be required to achieve it.

_____ _____
_____ _____
_____ _____
_____ _____
_____ _____
_____ _____

TIME INTERVAL REWARDS

To help you continue to practice your new eating behaviors and achieve your desired weight loss, you should reward yourself at set time intervals.

First determine your reward for successfully losing 4 to 12 pounds of weight each month. At the end of each month in which you achieve this goal, give yourself a reward greater in value than any you selected for achieving success at weekly intervals.

TASK NO. 37

List below your choice of rewards for:

1. First month

_____

_____

2. Second month

_____

_____

3. Third month

_____

_____

4. Fourth month

_____

_____

4. Determine Your Weight Goal

As you begin your weight loss program, take a close look at where you are now and where you will go in terms of your weight.

The graph on the following page permits you to visualize your progress toward your weight goal.

TASK NO. 38

Complete the following items on the graph on the following page:

1. Select on the weight scale the points which indicate both your present weight and your desired weight and circle them as shown.

2. If you do not know your desired weight, you can refer to any standard table or consult your physician.

3. Draw a horizontal line from your desired weight across the graph (see solid line).

4. At the end of the first week, weigh yourself and put a dot on vertical line 1 at the appropriate weight line (see graph). Repeat each subsequent week.

5. Record your weight *loss* (actual number of pounds lost) on the horizontal line where your new weight meets the number of the week you are in on the program.

WEIGHT LOSS GRAPH

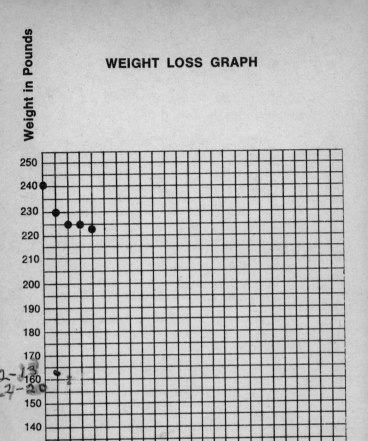

Weight in Pounds

Weeks on Weight Loss Program

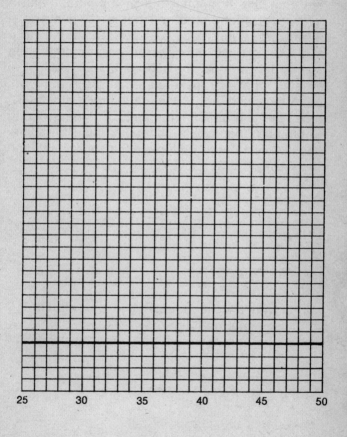

25   30   35   40   45   50

5. Long-Term Rewards

THE CONTRACT

You may find it helpful to sign a contract with a relative or friend who will agree to give you a reward when you reach your desired weight. Have a discussion with this person and determine an appropriate reward for achieving your goal. It is essential that you make sure that the reward will be forthcoming, and if you are in doubt about this, it can be held by a neutral party. The person with whom you negotiate a contract should be someone who is sincerely interested in your health and well-being.

TASK NO. 39

If you choose to enter into a contract, complete the following:

CONTRACT

I, _____ , agree

to give to _____

a _____
        (monetary or other reward)
when you reach your desired weight of
_____ pounds.

Signed
_____

Witnessed
_____

Date
_____

THE AGREEMENT

You can also make a pact with another person in which you both agree to begin this weight loss program.

Each of you can put up a certain sum of money or gift item to be given to the one who is first to reach his desired weight. If you tend to be competitive, this kind of agreement may appeal to you.

TASK NO. 40

If you wish you can make the following agreement:

AGREEMENT

I, _____ and

I, _____ ,

each agree to forfeit $ _____ to the

other, if I do not lose _____ pounds

by _____
                    (date)

Signed _____

Signed _____

Witnessed _____

Date _____

6. Consolidating Your New Eating Behaviors

You are now familiar with our weight loss program. By focusing your efforts on new and more constructive eating behavior, you will be able to reach your desired weight and collect your rewards. These rewards are important, but they are secondary to the sense of accomplishment and satisfaction that you will feel for having learned your new eating behavior. This feeling of self-mastery will be strengthened as you continue to practice them and maintain your normal weight. It is important for you to weigh yourself on a weekly basis and to follow your progress on your graph.

You should strive to remain within 2 to 3 pounds of the desired weight you have achieved. If you fall below this level, do not give up your newly acquired eating patterns. Instead, just add controlled amounts of food to your menu models.

You may devise new rewards for maintaining your desired weight. Suggested intervals for these rewards are every three to six months.

When you have reached your goal, your primary emphasis should continue to be on your new eating behavior. The more you practice, the more ingrained and automatic this behavior will become.

Remember, as in tennis, if you develop a sound stroke, you can develop a winning game.

7. Looking Forward

Previously your weight goal has been elusive. We believe that in following this book you can learn the behaviors necessary to bring about and maintain normal weight.

For much of your life, you experienced the disastrous consequences of being overweight. You should begin to enjoy the pleasant consequences of normal weight. You are ready to enjoy not only a new sense of physical well-being and a greater sense of attractiveness to others, but, equally important, you will like yourself better. You will have a sense of mastery and control as well as pride and self-confidence. These feelings about yourself will lead you to new enriching involvements and greater achievement in your other endeavors.

This is just the beginning of a new healthier and happier you!

ABOUT THE AUTHORS

Walter H. Fanburg, M.D.

Princeton University, A.B.
Tulane University School of Medicine, M.D.
Psychiatric training at Tulane University School of
  Medicine
Diplomate of the American Board of Psychiatry
  and Neurology
Member of the American Psychiatric Association

Bernard M. Snyder, M.D.

Franklin and Marshall College, A.B.
Woodrow Wilson Fellow, Harvard University Grad-
  uate School
Columbia University College of Physicians and
  Surgeons, M.D.
Psychiatric training at Yale University School of
  Medicine
Diplomate of the American Board of Psychiatry
  and Neurology
Member of the American Psychiatric Association

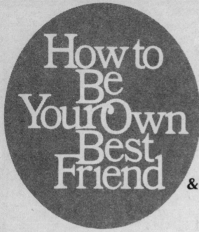